BLADDER DISEASES

UNDERSTANDING TYPES, CAUSES, DIAGNOSIS, TREATMENT, AND MANAGEMENT

DR. J.P JUDE

Table of Contents

CHAPTER ONE

INTRODUCTION

Bladder illnesses are a group of disorders that impact the bladder's overall health, structure, and function. These disorders can cause a variety of symptoms and problems. As an essential component of the urinary system, the bladder keeps and excretes urine from the body, regulates fluid balance, and eliminates waste.

Recognizing bladder disorders' causes, symptoms, risk factors, diagnostic techniques, and available treatments is essential to understanding them. Bladder disorders can have a major impact on a person's quality of life, overall health, and ability to urinate. These conditions can range from benign conditions like bladder stones and urinary tract infections (UTIs) to more serious conditions like interstitial cystitis and bladder cancer.

The purpose of this introduction is to give a general review of common bladder illnesses while emphasizing their significance for individual, public, and clinical practice. People can take proactive measures to improve bladder health, optimize treatment outcomes, and address bladder disorders by increasing awareness, encouraging early detection, and encouraging proactive management.

In order to enhance bladder health and general well-being, we will explore the architecture and function of the bladder, various bladder disorders, risk factors, signs and symptoms, diagnostic evaluations, treatment modalities, prevention techniques, and self-care practices throughout this exploration.

Continue reading to find out more about bladder illnesses, how they affect daily living and health, and how proactive management and working with healthcare professionals are crucial for achieving the best possible bladder health and quality of life.

Bladder's Anatomy and Function

The lower abdomen's bladder, a crucial organ, is in charge of holding and eliminating pee from the body. Recognizing its importance for the urinary system and general health requires an understanding of its architecture and function. An outline of the anatomy and function of the bladder is provided here:

The Bladder's Anatomy

Bladder Wall: The bladder's tissue is divided into multiple layers, which include:

Urothelium (Inner Lining): An adapted epithelial lining that expands to hold pee and stops urine from seeping into the bladder wall.

Muscular Layer (Detrusor Muscle): A substantial layer of smooth muscle that relaxes to allow the bladder to fill with pee and contracts to release urine during urination.

Submucosa: The bladder wall's supporting and shielding layer of connective tissue.

The outermost layer that gives the bladder extra support and defense is called the serosa or adventitia.

The urethra, which is a tube-like structure that transports urine from the bladder to the outside of the body, is connected to the bladder via the bladder neck.

What the Bladder Does:

The bladder serves the following main purposes:

Storage of Urine: The kidneys' output of urine is held in the bladder until it is opportune to empty it. The bladder may hold different volumes of pee because of its capacity to expand and shrink.

Urine Expulsion (Voiding): Sensory nerve fibers in the bladder wall notify the brain when the bladder reaches a specific capacity, signaling the urge to urinate. Urine can be released from the bladder through the urethra when the external urethral sphincter is willingly relaxed and the detrusor muscle is contracted.

Urine Composition: Waste products, toxins, and extra fluid that the kidneys have filtered out are all present in urine, which is why the inner lining of the bladder makes mucus to shield the bladder wall from any potential damage.

Mechanisms of Control:

The intricate interaction of muscles, nerves, and reflexes is necessary for proper bladder control in order to preserve urinary continence and regulate the frequency and timing of urination:

Bladder Muscles (Detrusor Muscle): The detrusor muscle helps with urine storage and ejection by contracting and relaxing.

Internal and external urethral sphincters: these muscles regulate how much urine exits the bladder. While the external sphincter can be deliberately managed to start or stop urination, the internal sphincter opens spontaneously when the bladder is full.

Nerves: When the bladder fills and fills to capacity, sensory nerve fibers in the bladder wall notify the brain. In order to regulate the flow of pee and synchronize the timing of urination, the brain reacts by sending signals back to the bladder and sphincters.

By retaining fluid balance, eliminating waste from the body, and storing and releasing urine, the bladder is an essential component of the urinary system. People can better understand the bladder's role in preserving urine continence, promoting general health, and averting diseases and disorders of the bladder by learning about its structure and function.

Watch this space to learn about different bladder illnesses, how they affect bladder function, and how to keep your bladder healthy and happy.

Bladder illnesses are a broad category of disorders that impact the structure, function, and general health of the bladder, resulting in a range of symptoms and problems. For the best possible management, early diagnosis, and proper treatment, it is imperative to understand the many forms of bladder disorders. The following are a few typical kinds of bladder diseases:

1. UTIs, or urinary tract infections:

Bacterial infections known as UTIs can impact any area of the urinary tract, encompassing the kidneys (pyelonephritis), urethra (urethritis), and bladder (cystitis). Symptoms of urinary tract infections (UTIs) include pain or burning when urinating, bloody or murky urine, and pelvic pain.

2. Urinary calculi, or bladder stones:

Bladder stones are mineral deposits that occur in the bladder as a result of minerals crystallizing and urine becoming concentrated. Urinary tract infections, bloody urine, trouble urinating, lower abdomen pain, and frequent urination are some of the symptoms that these stones can cause.

3. Cancer of the Bladder:

Description: Uncontrollably growing abnormal cells in the bladder lining cause bladder cancer. Adenocarcinoma, squamous cell carcinoma, and urothelial carcinoma are common forms of bladder cancer. Blood in the urine, frequent urination, pain during urination, and pelvic or lower back pain are possible symptoms.

4. Bladder Pain Syndrome/Interstitial Cystitis (IC/BPS):

The symptoms of IC/BPS, a chronic illness, include nocturia, urgency, and frequency of urination in the bladder. Although the precise origin of IC/BPS is uncertain, it may be related to anomalies in the bladder's protective lining or bladder lining inflammation.

5. Bladder overactivity (OAB):

The symptoms of OAB include frequent urination, nocturia, and an unexpected, overwhelming urge to urinate. It could be brought on by nerve injury, involuntary bladder contractions, or other underlying medical issues.

6. Blockage of the Bladder Outlet:

Bladder outlet occlusion is a condition in which the bladder's ability to empty its contents freely is impeded by an obstruction. Bladder stones, malignancies, UTIs, prostate enlargement in men, and pelvic organ prolapse in women are a few possible causes. Urinary retention, poor urine flow, difficulties beginning, and incomplete bladder emptying are some symptoms.

7. Bladder Neurogenic:

The term "neurogenic bladder" refers to bladder dysfunction brought on by a neurological condition or trauma that impairs bladder control. Urinary incontinence, retention, and bladder dysfunction can result from diseases such multiple sclerosis, stroke, Parkinson's disease, spinal cord injuries, and other disorders that interfere with nerve communication between the bladder and brain.

8. Radiation Cystitis:

Radiation therapy for pelvic malignancies can induce inflammation and damage to the bladder lining, which is known as radiation cystitis. Urine symptoms can include burning or pain when urinating, urgency, frequent urination, blood in the urine, and spasms in the bladder.

Bladder diseases impact people differently according to their age, gender, health status, and lifestyle variables. They can also differ in kind, severity, and underlying causes. Awareness of the warning signs and symptoms of bladder disorders, proper diagnostic testing, and customized treatment planning can help people effectively manage bladder conditions, improve their ability to urinate, and improve their overall quality of life.

To prevent bladder disorders, promote bladder health, and support good urine continence throughout life, it is imperative to consult with healthcare professionals, maintain regular medical check-ups, practice preventative measures, and adopt healthy lifestyle behaviors.

CHAPTER TWO

Reasons and Danger Elements

Preventive measures, early detection, and efficient therapy of bladder disorders all depend on an understanding of the risk factors and causes of these conditions. Below is a summary of the risk factors and prevalent causes of the many bladder diseases:

1. UTIs, or urinary tract infections:

Reasons:

germs: The most frequent cause of urinary tract infections (UTIs) is bacterial infection, usually caused by Escherichia coli (E. coli) germs that enter the urinary tract from the digestive tract.

Gender: Because women have shorter urethras, which provide germs greater access to the bladder, they are more likely to get UTIs.

Sexual Activity: Having sex might cause bacteria to enter the urine system.

UTI Risk: The use of a urinary catheter carries a higher risk of infection.

An increased risk of urinary tract infections (UTIs) can result from structural abnormalities in the urinary system.

Menopause: The environment of the urinary system can change due to hormonal changes during menopause, which raises the risk of UTIs.

2. Urinary calculi, or bladder stones:

Reasons:

Mineral Imbalance: Stone formation and mineral crystallization can result from concentrated urine.

Bladder Outlet Obstruction: Bladder stones can develop as a result of obstructions in the urinary tract or bladder.

Hazardous Elements

Age: Dietary variables, decreased bladder emptying, and dehydration all put older persons at higher risk.

Gender: Compared to women, men are more likely to get bladder stones.

Medical Conditions: Risk factors include metabolic abnormalities, bladder diverticula, and urinary tract infections.

Diet: Diets heavy in protein and salt have been linked to the development of stones.

3. Cancer of the Bladder:

Reasons:

Use of Tobacco: The biggest risk factor for bladder cancer is smoking.

Chemical Exposure: There is an increased risk associated with exposure to specific chemicals, including arsenic and chemicals used in the leather, rubber, and textile industries.

Chronic Bladder Inflammation: Bladder cancer risk is raised by persistent bladder irritation and inflammation.

Genetic Factors: Genetic mutations and family history can put a person at risk for bladder cancer.

Hazardous Elements

Age: The majority of cases are diagnosed in adults over 55, and the risk rises with age.

Gender: Bladder cancer is more common in men than in women.

Race: Compared to Asian and African Americans, Caucasians are more vulnerable.

Occupational Exposures: There may be a higher risk in some jobs involving chemical exposure.

Chronic Bladder Infections: The risk may be raised by recurrent or persistent bladder infections.

4. Bladder Pain Syndrome/Interstitial Cystitis (IC/BPS):

Reasons:

Unknown: Although the precise origin of IC/BPS is unknown, it may be related to pelvic floor dysfunction, immunological reactions, or bladder inflammation.

Hazardous Elements

Gender: Compared to men, women are more likely to acquire IC/BPS.

Age: As people age, their risk increases.

Other Chronic illnesses: Irritable bowel syndrome, fibromyalgia, and chronic fatigue syndrome are a few examples of chronic pain illnesses that may coexist with IC/BPS.

5. Bladder overactivity (OAB):

Reasons:

Muscle Dysfunction: OAB may result from the bladder muscles' hyperactivity or spasms.

Nerve Damage: Disorders such as diabetes, multiple sclerosis, and Parkinson's disease can cause damage to the nerves, which can impair bladder function.

Hazardous Elements

Age: As people age, their risk increases.

Gender: OAB is more common in women than in men.

Medical Conditions: Risk factors include diabetes, neurological diseases, and bladder infections.

Numerous variables, including as bacterial infections, mineral imbalances, chemical exposures, genetic predispositions, lifestyle decisions, and underlying medical disorders, can contribute to bladder diseases. In order to limit risk, manage symptoms, and maximize bladder health, prevention, early identification, and focused therapies are contingent upon an understanding of the causes and risk factors associated with bladder disorders.

Regular medical check-ups, healthy lifestyle choices, preventive care, and prompt medical attention for bladder-related symptoms or concerns can all help people lower their risk of bladder diseases, support bladder function, and improve their general health.

Symptoms and Indications

Understanding the telltale signs and symptoms of bladder disorders is essential for prompt diagnosis, effective treatment, and early detection. The following summarizes the typical indications and symptoms of the several bladder diseases:

1. UTIs, or urinary tract infections:

Strong urge to urinate more frequently than usual is known as frequent urination.

Burning or Painful Sensation: Burning or painful feeling during urinating.

Bloody or hazy urine: Urine can seem hazy, dark, or bleeding.

Lower abdominal or pelvic pain is referred to as pelvic pain.

Urgency: An abrupt, strong need to go to the bathroom.

Fever or Chills: Weariness, fever, and chills could all be signs of a more serious infection.

2. Urinary calculi, or bladder stones:

Chronic pain in the lower abdomen or pelvis is referred to as lower abdominal pain.

Urination that hurts: Urinating that hurts or causes discomfort.

Increased frequency of urinating is known as frequent urination.

Urination Difficulties: Inability to initiate or sustain a continuous stream of urine.

Bloody Urine: Blood can appear in urine and take on a pink, red, or brown color.

3. Cancer of the Bladder:

Hematuria, or blood in the urine, is defined as either visible blood in the urine or pee that looks rusty or dark.

Urination that hurts: Urinating that hurts or causes discomfort.

Increased frequency of urinating is known as frequent urination.

Back or Pelvic Pain: Soreness in the sides, lower back, or pelvis.

Urinary Urgency: An unexpected, strong need to urinate.

4. Bladder Pain Syndrome/Interstitial Cystitis (IC/BPS):

Chronic pelvic pain refers to ongoing discomfort in the pelvis or bladder.

Increased urine frequency, especially nocturia (nighttime urination).

Urinary Urgency: An unexpected, strong need to urinate.

Painful Intercourse: Any discomfort or pain experienced during a sexual encounter.

Bladder pressure or pain that becomes worse as the bladder fills up is known as painful bladder syndrome.

5. Bladder overactivity (OAB):

Urinary urgency: an intense, unexpected need to go to the bathroom.

Having to urinate more frequently than usual is known as frequent urination.

Urinating in the middle of the night, or nocturia.

Urge Incontinence: the uncontrollably sudden need to urinate that results in the loss of urine.

6. Blockage of the Bladder Outlet:

Urination Difficulty: Difficulty launching the pee stream.

Weak pee Stream: A pee stream with less force or volume.

Feeling that the bladder is not entirely emptied after urinating is known as incomplete emptying.

Urinary Retention: Having trouble passing urine, which results in discomfort or a full feeling in the bladder.

Numerous indications and symptoms, from pelvic pain and blood in the urine to urinary discomfort and behavioral changes, can indicate the presence of bladder illnesses. Accurate diagnosis, suitable therapy, and management of bladder diseases depend on the recognition of these symptoms and prompt medical evaluation.

It's important to speak with medical specialists if you have any persistent or worrisome symptoms pertaining to bladder health so they can provide you with a thorough evaluation, diagnosis, and individualized treatment plan based on your needs. Improving general well-being, minimizing problems, and maximizing bladder health all depend on early detection, timely action, and continuing care.

Diagnostic Assessment

A thorough method is used in the diagnostic evaluation of bladder disorders in order to determine the underlying cause, validate the diagnosis, and create a suitable treatment strategy. To assess bladder function, find problems, and inform treatment choices, medical professionals may combine clinical evaluations, laboratory testing, imaging studies, and specialized procedures. An outline of typical diagnostic tests for bladder disorders is provided below:

1. Medical Background and Physical Assessment:

Patient History: Information on medications, lifestyle choices, medical history, and family history of bladder disorders can be gathered to help determine the severity and possible origin of bladder issues.

CHAPTER THREE

Physical Examination: To examine bladder function, spot anomalies, and rule out other medical issues, a comprehensive physical examination may involve neurological testing, pelvic exams for women, and abdominal probing.

2. Analyzing urine:

Urine Sample Analysis: A urinalysis is a frequent diagnostic test that looks for abnormalities in the urine, such as blood, protein, sugar, or other substances that may indicate bladder or urinary tract problems, as well as indicators of infection.

3. Culture of Urine:

Urine cultures can be used to identify the particular bacteria causing an infection and to establish the best course of therapy for an infection, if a urinary tract infection (UTI) is suspected.

4. Imaging Research:

Ultrasound: To detect anomalies such bladder stones, tumors, or structural abnormalities, an abdominal or pelvic ultrasound employs sound waves to create images of the bladder, kidneys, and urinary system.

Computed Tomography (CT) Scan: A CT scan can detect tumors, stones, inflammation, or other abnormalities by providing precise cross-sectional images of the bladder, kidneys, and surrounding structures.

Magnetic Resonance Imaging (MRI): An MRI is a diagnostic tool that combines radio waves and magnetic fields to produce comprehensive images of the pelvic area and bladder. It is especially helpful in the evaluation of soft tissue anomalies, tumors, and bladder cancer.

5. Cystoscopy:

Direct Visualization: Cystoscopy is a minimally invasive treatment in which the bladder and urethra are punctured to allow for the visual inspection of the bladder lining, the identification of anomalies, and, if required, the removal of tissue samples (biopsy).

6. Tests for Urodynamics:

Bladder Function Assessment: In order to diagnose diseases such as overactive bladder (OAB), bladder outlet obstruction, and neurogenic bladder, urodynamic testing assesses bladder function, urine flow, and pressure changes in the bladder and urethra during bladder filling and emptying.

7. autopsy

Tissue Sample Analysis: A biopsy may be necessary to remove tissue samples from the bladder lining for microscopic analysis in order to diagnose bladder cancer, inflammation, or other pathological disorders if abnormalities are found during a cystoscopy or imaging tests.

Bladder disease diagnostic evaluations are customized based on patient symptoms, medical history, and clinical results to guarantee correct diagnosis and suitable treatment. The identification of bladder diseases, the direction of treatment decisions, and the enhancement of patient outcomes are contingent upon the timely detection, thorough assessment, and specialized testing.

It's critical to speak with medical professionals if you have ongoing or worrisome symptoms pertaining to your bladder's health so they can provide you with a comprehensive evaluation, diagnosis, and individualized treatment plan that is specific to your needs and situation. In order to manage bladder disorders, promote bladder health, and improve overall well-being, collaborative treatment, frequent follow-up, and continuous monitoring are crucial.

Methods of Therapy

Bladder disease treatment strategies are to reduce symptoms, treat underlying causes, avoid complications, enhance bladder function, and enhance overall quality of life. Depending on the particular bladder condition, the intensity of symptoms, the needs of each patient, and the outcome of early therapies, the treatment approach may change. An outline of popular methods for treating bladder problems is provided below:

1. UTIs, or urinary tract infections:

Antibiotic Therapy: By focusing on and getting rid of the causing bacteria, oral antibiotics are used to treat bacterial UTIs.

Pain Relieving Drugs: To ease the pain and discomfort brought on by UTIs, over-the-counter or prescription pain relievers may be advised.

Increased Fluid Intake: Water consumption promotes the body's natural healing process and aids in the removal of bacteria from the urinary tract.

2. Urinary calculi, or bladder stones:

Medical Expulsion Therapy: Drugs like potassium citrate that are meant to dissolve stones in the bladder can be used to treat small stones.

Surgical Removal: Cystolithapaxy, or open surgery, may be necessary to remove larger bladder stones or stones that do not respond to medication.

Fluid Intake: Drinking more water can help dissolve minor bladder stones and stop new ones from forming.

3. Cancer of the Bladder:

Surgery: To remove malignant tumors or the entire bladder, surgical techniques such as transurethral resection of bladder tumor (TURBT), partial cystectomy, or radical cystectomy may be used.

Chemotherapy: Drugs used in chemotherapy can be used either before or after surgery to reduce tumor size, eradicate cancer cells, or stop cancer from coming back.

Radiation therapy: Especially for non-invasive or advanced-stage bladder cancer, radiation therapy can be utilized to kill cancer cells or reduce tumors.

4. Bladder Pain Syndrome/Interstitial Cystitis (IC/BPS):

Bladder Instillations: To lessen inflammation, ease pain, and enhance bladder function, medications like heparin, lidocaine, or dimethyl sulfoxide (DMSO) may be injected directly into the bladder.

Oral Medications: Pentosan polysulfate sodium (Elmiron), antihistamines, tricyclic antidepressants, and other drugs may be recommended to treat bladder symptoms and alleviate discomfort and inflammation.

Pain Management: To treat persistent pelvic pain related to IC/BPS, medicines for nerve discomfort, muscle relaxants, and pain relievers may be utilized.

5. Bladder overactivity (OAB):

Bladder Training: Behavioral therapies, which include timed voiding schedules and bladder training, can help decrease urgency in the urine and lengthen the intervals between urinal trips.

Exercises for the Pelvic Floor: Kegel exercises and training for the muscles supporting the bladder help strengthen the pelvic floor, increase bladder support, and improve urine control.

Medication: To relax the bladder muscles, lessen bladder spasms, and manage urine symptoms, doctors may prescribe beta-3 agonists, anticholinergic or antimuscarinic medicines, and other prescription medications.

6. Blockage of the Bladder Outlet:

Catheterization: In order to reduce urinary retention and empty the bladder, a temporary or permanent catheterization may be necessary.

Medication: To relax the muscles in the bladder neck, enhance urine flow, and lessen obstruction, doctors may prescribe alpha-blockers, 5-alpha reductase inhibitors, and other drugs.

Surgery: To eliminate obstructions and restore normal urine flow, surgical treatments such as transurethral resection of the prostate (TURP), prostatectomy, or bladder neck incision may be carried out.

In order to guarantee the best possible results, symptom relief, and an enhanced quality of life, treatment strategies for bladder disorders are customized to each patient's symptoms, diagnosis, and unique bladder circumstances. In order to manage bladder disorders, promote bladder health, and improve overall well-being, collaborative treatment, multidisciplinary interventions, regular monitoring, and continuing support are crucial.

It is crucial to speak with medical specialists if you or someone you know is having problems or symptoms connected to the bladder. They can provide a thorough assessment, a diagnosis, and a customized treatment plan based on each patient's needs, preferences, and condition. Sustaining good bladder function and well-being and effectively managing bladder diseases requires early intervention, prompt treatment, and patient-centered care.

Control and Assistive Healthcare

For people with bladder illnesses, management and supportive care are essential to maximizing bladder health, controlling symptoms, and improving quality of life. An all-encompassing strategy that incorporates behavioral therapy, supportive interventions, lifestyle changes, and medicinal treatments can help people manage bladder issues, reduce discomfort, and enhance their general quality of life. An outline of supportive care and management approaches for bladder illnesses is provided below:

1. Medical Surveillance and Aftercare:

Frequent Check-ups: Arrange for routine medical examinations with healthcare professionals to keep an eye on bladder function, assess the efficacy of treatments, and modify treatment regimens as necessary.

Diagnostic Tests: To keep an eye on the health of your bladder, spot recurrences, or spot new changes, get periodic diagnostic tests such cystoscopies, imaging investigations, and urinalyses.

2. Management of Medication:

Adherence to Medication: To control bladder function, manage symptoms, and avoid complications, take prescription drugs as instructed by medical professionals.

Side Effect Management: Notify medical professionals of any negative drug reactions or concerns so they can make the necessary modifications, choose a different course of action, or implement supportive care measures.

3. Behavioral Therapies and Modifications to Lifestyle:

Use bladder training methods to lengthen the intervals between bathroom visits, lessen urgency when urinating, and enhance bladder control.

Exercises for the Pelvic Floor: Perform regular pelvic floor muscular exercises (Kegels) to support bladder function, strengthen pelvic muscles, and improve urine control.

Dietary Modifications: To lessen bladder symptoms and irritation, adopt an acidic diet and stay away from foods that are acidic, spicy, caffeine, alcohol, and artificial sweeteners.

Fluid management: To prevent frequent urination or irritation of the bladder, stay well-hydrated throughout the day by drinking lots of water.

4. Physical therapy for the pelvic floor:

Specialized Therapy: For individualized treatment plans, exercises, and procedures to address pelvic floor dysfunction, urine incontinence, and pelvic pain related to bladder diseases, consult pelvic floor physical therapists.

5. Counseling and Encouragement:

Patient education: To arm yourself with knowledge and make wise decisions, look for information, resources, and educational materials on bladder problems, treatment options, self-management techniques, and lifestyle suggestions.

Support Groups: To connect with others, exchange stories, get support, and pick up coping mechanisms from peers and medical professionals, join support groups, online forums, or neighborhood organizations devoted to bladder health.

Counseling Services: To address emotional, psychological, or social concerns associated to bladder disorders, chronic pain, lifestyle modifications, and coping with bladder-related challenges, take into consideration counseling, psychological support, or therapy.

6. Innovative Interventions and Therapies:

Surgical Procedures: If you have a problem that doesn't improve with conservative treatment, needs intervention, or presents a serious risk to your health, talk to your doctor about your options, concerns, advantages, and alternatives before undergoing surgery.

Advanced Therapies: Under the supervision of qualified healthcare professionals, investigate cutting-edge treatments for neurogenic bladder diseases, urine retention, and refractory bladder conditions, such as neuromodulation, botox injections, bladder augmentation, or nerve stimulation.

Bladder disease management and supportive care require a comprehensive strategy that emphasizes patient empowerment, lifestyle modifications, symptom control, and tailored treatment. Bladder disorders can be effectively managed by patients using a combination of medical treatments, behavioral therapies, lifestyle modifications, and supportive interventions. This can reduce symptoms, improve bladder function, and improve overall quality of life.

It's critical to speak with medical professionals, specialists, or support services if you or someone you know is experiencing symptoms, worries, or difficulties related to the bladder. They can provide a thorough evaluation, a diagnosis, treatment planning, and ongoing support that is customized to each patient's needs, preferences, and circumstances. Personalized therapies, patient-centered care, and collaborative care are essential for effectively managing bladder disorders, encouraging bladder health, and bolstering overall well-being throughout the healthcare process.

Difficulties and Outlook

Bladder disease complications and prognoses differ based on the particular ailment, degree of severity, underlying causes, and response to treatment. Certain bladder disorders can be treated with proper treatments, making them readily manageable, but others can result in chronic conditions, recurrent symptoms, or potential complications that need to be monitored continuously, treated with modifications, or treated with additional interventions. The prognosis and possible complications for common bladder disorders are summarized as follows:

1. UTIs, or urinary tract infections:

Problems:

Recurrent Infections: UTIs that occur frequently or repeatedly may be a sign of underlying problems such kidney infections, abnormalities of the bladder, or obstructions of the urinary tract.

Damage to the Kidneys: If left untreated or severed, urinary tract infections (UTIs) can cause kidney damage, pyelonephritis, or sepsis, a potentially fatal systemic infection.

Forecast:

Positive: Most UTIs are treatable with little long-term side effects when diagnosed promptly, treated with the right antibiotics, and prevented.

2. Urinary calculi, or bladder stones:

Problems:

Urinary blockage brought on by large bladder stones might result in infection, renal injury, or urine retention.

Recurrence: Bladder stones may return if underlying causes are not treated or modified in diet.

Forecast:

Good to Fair: The majority of bladder stones can be managed or treated with drugs, non-invasive procedures, or surgical interventions, depending on the size, nature, and location of the stones.

CHAPTER FOUR

3. Cancer of the Bladder:

Problems:

Cancer Spread: Bladder cancer has the potential to metastasis, or spread, to surrounding tissues, lymph nodes, or other organs. This can result in advanced disease stages, more difficult treatment options, and a lower chance of survival.

Recurrence: Following therapy, bladder cancer may return, necessitating continued surveillance, monitoring, and maybe retreatment.

Forecast:

Variable: The prognosis for bladder cancer is contingent upon the cancer's stage, grade, kind, location, and extent, as well as the patient's age, general health, and therapy response. Increased prognosis and survival rates can be achieved with prompt discovery, thorough treatment planning, and early interventions.

4. Bladder Pain Syndrome/Interstitial Cystitis (IC/BPS):

Problems:

Chronic Pain: Prolonged pelvic pain, bladder pain, or discomfort can have a serious negative influence on everyday functioning, emotional health, and quality of life.

Decreased Bladder Capacity: Urinary urgency, frequent urination, nocturia, and reduced bladder capacity can all result from severe cases of IC/BPS.

Forecast:

Chronic Condition: In order to control symptoms, lessen pain, enhance bladder function, and enhance quality of life, individuals with IC/BPS may need to make lifestyle adjustments and utilize multimodal therapy techniques.

5. Bladder overactivity (OAB):

Problems:

Decreased Quality of Life: The frequency, urgency, and incontinence of urination can have a major influence on everyday activities, social interactions, and emotional health.

Sleep disturbances: Nocturia, or the urinating of night, can cause sleep disturbances that result in exhaustion, sleeplessness, and a lower quality of life.

Forecast:

Handleable Condition: To control symptoms, improve bladder function, and improve overall well-being, OAB is a manageable condition that can be treated with a variety of methods, including behavioral therapy, lifestyle modifications, and medical interventions.

It is crucial to comprehend the prognosis and possible problems linked to bladder disorders in order to make well-informed decisions and to plan treatments and continue with continuing care. It is possible to reduce risks, enhance treatment outcomes, and promote bladder health and general well-being by implementing early diagnosis, prompt intervention, thorough care, frequent monitoring, and adherence to treatment guidelines.

It's critical to speak with medical professionals, specialists, or support services if you or someone you know is experiencing symptoms, worries, or difficulties related to the bladder. They can provide a comprehensive assessment, a customized treatment plan, and ongoing support that is suited to the needs, preferences, and circumstances of each patient. The key to successfully managing bladder disorders, maintaining bladder health, and supporting overall well-being throughout the healthcare journey is collaborative care, proactive management, and patient-centered approaches.

Avoidance and Mitigation of Risks

Maintaining bladder health, lowering the prevalence of bladder disorders, and lowering the risk of consequences from bladder conditions all depend heavily on prevention and risk reduction techniques. People can safeguard their bladder, maximize urine function, and improve overall well-being by embracing good lifestyle behaviors, taking preventive actions, and being aware of risk factors. An outline of risk mitigation techniques and preventive measures for bladder health is provided below:

1. Sustain a Healthy Fluid Intake and Remain Hydrated:

Sufficient Hydration: To stay hydrated, support urine function, and remove toxins from the urinary system, drink a lot of water throughout the day.

Limit Bladder Irritants: To lessen bladder irritation and any associated symptoms, cut back on your intake of substances that can irritate your bladder, such as caffeine, alcohol, carbonated beverages, spicy food, artificial sweeteners, and acidic foods.

2. Adopt Good Urinary and Hygiene Practices:

Personal Hygiene: To lower your risk of urinary tract infections (UTIs), practice good personal hygiene by washing frequently, wiping after using the restroom from front to back, and keeping your genital area clean.

Urinary Habits: Lower your risk of urinary tract infections (UTIs) and bladder infections by completely emptying your bladder on a regular basis, avoiding holding onto pee for extended periods of time.

3. Have a Healthy Lifestyle and Balanced Diet:

Nutritional Balance: To promote general health, immunological function, and bladder wellness, eat a diet rich in fruits, vegetables, whole grains, lean meats, and healthy fats.

Weight management: To lower the risk of bladder disorders, urine incontinence, and pelvic floor dysfunction, maintain a healthy weight by regular exercise, a balanced diet, and portion control.

4. Exercises for the Pelvic Floor and Bladder Training:

Exercises for the Pelvic Floor: Regularly perform Kegels to strengthen the pelvic muscles, boost bladder support, improve urine control, and lower the chance of urinary incontinence.

Use bladder training strategies to gradually increase the intervals between urinations in order to enhance bladder control, lessen urgency, and lengthen the duration between bathroom visits.

5. Steer Clear of Tobacco and Reduce Chemical Exposures:

Tobacco Cessation: Give up smoking and keep yourself away from secondhand smoke to lower your chance of bladder cancer, chronic inflammation of the bladder, and other bladder-related issues.

Chemical Safety: Use safety precautions, adhere to safety regulations, and consult a professional before handling hazardous materials to reduce exposure to toxic chemicals, hazardous materials, and environmental pollutants at home or at work.

6. Frequent medical screenings and check-ups:

Routine Examinations: To monitor bladder health, identify early indicators of bladder disorders, and obtain prompt interventions, schedule routine medical check-ups, pelvic exams, and urological screenings with healthcare providers.

Screening Tests: To detect any bladder abnormalities or conditions, follow recommendations from your healthcare practitioner and based on your age, family history, risk factors, and medical history, get recommended screening tests such as imaging investigations, cystoscopy, and urinalysis.

7. Handle Medications and Chronic Conditions:

Chronic Condition Management: Lower the risk of bladder problems and urine dysfunction by managing chronic illnesses such diabetes, hypertension, obesity, and neurological disorders through multidisciplinary treatment, regular monitoring, medication management, and lifestyle changes.

Medication Review: To discover potential bladder irritants, interactions, or side effects that may alter urine function, bladder health, or raise the risk of bladder-related diseases, review prescription pharmaceuticals, over-the-counter medications, and supplements with healthcare specialists on a frequent basis.

Bladder health, urinary wellness, and general well-being all depend heavily on prevention and risk reduction. People can take proactive measures to preserve good urine function throughout their lives, lower their risk of bladder disorders, and take proactive management of their bladder health by implementing these methods into their daily routines, adopting educated lifestyle choices, and getting early medical guidance.

It is crucial to speak with medical professionals, urologists, or specialists if you or someone you know is worried about bladder-related symptoms, risks, or preventive measures. They can provide individualized advice, suggestions, and support based on each person's needs, preferences, and circumstances. In order to support overall well-being throughout the healthcare journey and to promote bladder health and avoid bladder illnesses, proactive management, collaborative care, and patient-centered approaches are essential.

Summary

To sum up, bladder health is critical to general health, life satisfaction, and day-to-day functioning. In order to maximize bladder function and maintain overall health, bladder disorders require thorough evaluation, prompt diagnosis, targeted therapies, and continuous care. These diseases can have a substantial influence on an individual's physical, mental, and social aspects of life.

People are better equipped to make educated decisions, adopt good living habits, practice preventative techniques, and seek prompt medical attention when necessary when they are aware of the anatomy, function, signs, symptoms, risk factors, and preventive actions connected to bladder illnesses. One can lower the risk of bladder issues, minimize complications, and improve overall well-being throughout life by emphasizing bladder health, identifying any concerns, and acting pro-actively.

Effective management of bladder diseases, promotion of bladder health, and maintenance of optimal urinary function throughout the healthcare journey necessitate collaborative care, multidisciplinary approaches, patient-centered interventions, and ongoing support from healthcare professionals, specialists, and support services.

It's critical to speak with healthcare professionals, urologists, or specialists if you or someone you know is dealing with bladder-related symptoms, worries, or difficulties in order to receive a thorough assessment, diagnosis, customized treatment plan, and supportive care catered to specific requirements, preferences, and conditions. Individuals can manage bladder disorders, preserve urinary wellness, and enhance overall quality of life for a healthier and happier future by cooperating, remaining informed, and placing a high priority on bladder health.

THE END

www.ingramcontent.com/pod-product-compliance
Lightning Source LLC
Chambersburg PA
CBHW061729250726
48657CB00002B/844